The DASH Diet for Weight Loss

The Ultimate Beginner DASH Diet Guide for Weight Loss, Lower Blood Pressure, and Better Health Including Delicious DASH Diet Recipes

Ella Marie

Table of Contents

Introduction

I want to thank you and congratulate you for downloading the book *"The Dash Diet."*

This book contains proven steps and strategies on how to lower your salt intake, improve your health, and enjoy great food.

If you have ever had symptoms that led to doctor's visits and medication, then you want to think about utilizing a diet like the DASH diet. Maybe your doctor has said you suffer from:

- A heart condition
- Hypertension
- Weight gain
- Diabetes or kidney disorders

I want you to know that this diet is a great option for you. The DASH diet is not just a diet, but a healthy alternative to transition your eating into a structured way to achieve optimal, long-term good health.

One problem that people run into over time is that they have all these great foods that they want to eat, but they don't realize that the salt content is so high that it's damaging their bodies.

The DASH diet is a way to rebalance your food so you can enjoy healthy options in everything you consume, that way you can ensure that you'll be around for a very long time! Because we worry so much about work stress and getting through the day, we sometimes fail to look at the amount of salt that's in the processed foods we eat. That's where the DASH diet comes in, because the DASH diet ensures that:

- you're eating healthy
- you're eating fresh
- you're consuming a lot of fruits and vegetables

Not only are you having a lot of fiber, but you're tying in a lot of protein through fresh meats like fish and other seafood, turkey, chicken, beef, and tofu.

The DASH diet is more than just weight loss; it's healthy eating, and that's why I want you to consider this diet as your healthy alternative. In this handy book, you'll learn about:

- What the DASH diet is and how it can help you
- The DASH diet in a step-by-step process
- The DASH diet to lose weight
- Combining foods and making adjustments, because part of dieting and part of changing your diet is making small adjustments with each and every meal
- Diet and exercise
- Different types of food that you can have that can help to lower your blood pressure
- Different types of meal plans that you can consider and sample diets in phases that might work for you
- Tips, pointers, and things that you may want to factor in as you switch over to the DASH diet

Remember one problem that people find along the way is that they want to eat things that are processed and have high salt content, and when they do that, they have to take a medication to bring the salt level down because their blood pressure is too high. That's why I want you to look at the DASH diet.

This natural alternative can not only have medicinal effects and great benefits, but it can also help to:

- Lower your blood pressure
- Address your diabetes issues
- Lose weight

Ultimately, I know the goal you have is to fix your sodium intake so you can stop taking blood pressure medicine and live a better life. The DASH diet will help you learn how to make adjustments to live a better lifestyle, and ultimately, that's the goal with this book.

Thanks again for purchasing this book, I hope you enjoy it!

CHAPTER 1
WHAT IS THE DASH DIET?

The DASH diet started out as a concept to help lower sodium and as a way to help people lose weight. The goal when it first began was to lower blood pressure. As the diet became more popular, it also became a healthier way of life. The DASH diet is basically a better way of targeting what you eat and ensuring that you are eating healthy meals by incorporating healthy, fresh foods. Because it ties things in such as healthy fruits, vegetables, nuts, seeds, whole grains, and fresh meat, you will find that not only is this diet tasty and enjoyable, but you'll wish that you had started it sooner!

The DASH diet is based on the letters in the word, which stand for Dietary Approaches to Stop and prevent Hypertension. This diet was set up as a step-by-step process to help you prolong your life by limiting the amount of salt that you consume. Instead of eating a lot of processed foods, you will focus on foods that are rich in vitamins, nutrients, and minerals such as calcium, potassium, and magnesium.

Getting Started

When you start the DASH diet, you want to keep track of how much you're eating as you work on portion control. You'll have different meal plans that you can have on a daily basis. The goal is to do the DASH diet a little bit at a time with each meal. You could start out using it for weight loss or just to lower your salt intake, practicing the diet and monitoring what you eat over the next two to four weeks.

After that, you want to keep it going. Have your blood pressure checked again so you can see how many points it has gone down; people who have tried the DASH diet have found that it really helps. The DASH diet can also help combat things such as heart disease, stroke, various forms of cancer, osteoporosis, and different levels of diabetes. The diet is able to target these different areas because you're changing the foods that you're eating. As you eat more fresh foods, such as your nuts, seafood, and greens, you're consuming healthier natural nutrients that are not processed like frozen foods.

How Can The Dash Diet Help Me?

The purpose of the DASH Diet is to:

- Change your eating habits
- Lower salt intake in your diet
- Reduce your blood pressure

Ultimately, this is done as you change what you eat. That's why it boils down to you, as you look at food in a new way.

What's In Your Processed Foods?

Someone may choose to eat a low-fat, frozen meal as a way of dieting. They sell these in different forms at the grocery store. The frozen meals may say on the packaging that they can help to lower your cholesterol, or they may say that they are low-fat and that they are a healthy alternative. However, when you look at the ingredients, you will likely see 700 to 800 milligrams of salt.

When you combine this with your other foods throughout the day, you may find that your salt level is so high that your feet are swelling up, you're retaining a lot of water, and your blood pressure is skyrocketing! That's where the DASH diet comes in. With the

DASH diet, because you're actually changing what you eat, those frozen foods are going right out the window! You can actually see changes right away because you're lowering salt consumption immediately.

As you incorporate more fresh and healthy foods, you'll start to see better benefits such as your skin clearing up and your digestion getting better, and you may find that your bowels actually move better. This is because you're incorporating healthy foods and a lot of fiber.

Fiber-Rich Foods

A person who is eating a frozen meal for dinner may only have that and no additional vegetables to accompany it. Or, if they do incorporate a salad, they may only be adding lettuce and tomatoes. The problem here is if you're not consuming rich nutrients that your body needs, you can have digestion issues such as constipation.

Protein Benefits

Other ways that you can help to change your eating habits with the DASH diet include how it will help you to incorporate fresh meat. Because you're using high levels of protein, it will trigger your body to expel extra salt and extra water. Protein helps to build muscle, and that's why you want to ensure you have a lot of it in your diet, as well as a lot of fiber to help you process it. That's why the DASH diet has included a lot of healthy vegetables and healthy fruits to ensure that you can easily digest your protein.

SAMPLE MEALS AND THE MINERALS IN THEM

When you look at a sample meal, it may be something like salmon for dinner. While you have salmon as your protein, you may want to have spinach and a side of sweet potatoes with that. Spinach contains calcium and iron, and your sweet potato contains calcium and different forms of magnesium and potassium. It's also rich in fiber, along with the spinach, which will aid in your digestion. The salmon will serve as your protein, and it's also a form of rich omega-3 fatty acids.

As you incorporate different nutrient-rich foods and proteins into your diet, this will enable your body to work the way that it should. You'll be better able to process foods, it will aid in digestion, and you can also enjoy the benefits of having a nutrient-rich diet, protein (which will build muscle), and lower fat.

Metabolic Effects

As salt comes off your diet, you're ridding your body of excess water, so you start to lose weight.

Protein also helps you build muscle in addition to lowering your bad fats and increasing your good, healthy fats. With this nutrient- and protein-rich diet, you will live a better life.

Low Salt Benefits

Lowering your salt intake can:

- lower your blood pressure
- reduce migraines or chronic sinus headaches
- lower your risk for diabetes
- reduce water retention

- reduce the risk for heart attacks and strokes
- reduce weight

As you continue with the DASH diet, you can actually develop a weight loss program. This can help you target the areas where you're having problems. You can combine the DASH diet with healthy snacks and your meals. For example, when you go to work or when you're at the gym, you can have healthy shakes or healthy snacks to ensure that you maintain the DASH diet all throughout the day.

Daily Salt Intake

As the DASH diet helps lower your salt intake, it increases your likelihood of having a healthier life that you can enjoy. Keep in mind that daily salt levels are usually about 3,500 milligrams or higher. They may even be 4,500 to 5,000 milligrams depending on what you're eating.

Consult A Physician

Your doctor may welcome the idea of you starting a diet like this. Have your doctor assess your sugar level, your blood pressure, your heart rate, and any medications that you may be on. That way, while using the diet, you'll be able to track your progress over time.

This book is divided into two parts, which are Phase 1, how to use the DASH diet on a daily basis, and Phase 2, how to incorporate exercise into your diet. I will also focus on having healthy foods and snacks, making daily adjustments, and establishing meal plans. So let's begin . . .

CHAPTER 2
WEIGHT LOSS: USING THE DASH DIET FOR WEIGHT LOSS AND EXERCISE

When you get ready to lose weight, you may make the mistake of trying to do it yourself. You may start out with the best of intentions; you find a diet plan that looks like it might work, load up on frozen, low-fat foods, and buy all of those protein bars. You may think you have a plan for success, and that's where you made the first mistake.

Food products may say they are healthy, but in reality, their salt level could be high without you realizing it. In the end, you may find that your blood pressure is still high or has gotten even higher! But because you saved time in the kitchen and your frozen meals tasted so good, you keep eating them!

Then, on top of that, you're constipated. That's a problem that happens when you go on a diet on your own or when you go on the wrong type of diet. When you get ready to use the DASH diet for weight loss, make sure the changes you make start in your refrigerator and your cabinet—by getting rid of those frozen and unhealthy foods.

Clean Out The Fridge And The Cabinets

Rid your cabinets of all processed foods. That means take out all of those TV dinners and protein bars. Limit the amount of alcohol and caffeine that you consume. Caffeine consumption does not necessarily affect blood pressure (aside from an initial spike), but you may want to limit your caffeine intake or keep it down because it can elevate your heart rate.

The DASH diet will help lose weight because it utilizes a lot of natural foods that don't have the preservatives and additives contained in processed and frozen foods. As you test it out to see whether or not your body will take to the diet, you may quickly realize that it's the type of diet you want to have for the rest of your life. You can incorporate a lot of fruits, vegetables, and good protein in the form of meat.

As you lower your risk for things like stroke, heart disease, and other ailments that are related to hypertension, you will see that the DASH diet quickly becomes something that is not just about losing weight but is about maintaining a healthy lifestyle.

The Dash Diet For Weight Loss

You're going to ideally have three full meals per day, and you will also have two to three small snacks in between. This diet is not about depriving you of food; you don't have to worry about starving or feeling like you can't eat. You'll be able to eat a lot of good, protein-rich foods. Let's look at some of the things that you can have in the diet so that you can make the appropriate changes.

Healthy Snacks

Nuts like almonds, peanuts, walnuts, cashews, and pecans can help ensure that you stay full throughout the day. You can also incorporate things like pumpkin seeds and edamame. If you get hungry and you want something sweet, your options are dried cranberries, raisins, bananas, apples, or any other piece of fruit. Don't worry; when you switch to Phase 2, you'll be able to have healthy nachos and potato skins or even make your own healthy snacks, like apple bran muffins and granola bars!

Keep in mind this is just a sample of some healthy snacks. This is not even incorporating the actual healthy foods that you can have once you achieve your optimal weight loss. That's why when you finish Phase 1, you want to stay on the DASH diet into Phase 2. When you switch over to the regular diet plan for life in Phase 2, the meals will get better, just like the snacks did. You'll be able to have things like bean dip, edamame hummus, and even whole wheat muffins.

Incorporating Exercise Into The DASH Diet

When you start exercising while you're on the DASH diet, the one thing that you may have to consider is how you're going to fuel your body. In the past, maybe your way of fueling your body was with a candy bar or a protein bar, but that may have been the reason you started packing on the pounds in the first place. With the DASH diet, you want to have appropriate foods that will help you during and after your workout.

For example, you want to have something that will fuel you for the workout and give you energy, which can come from proteins and carbs. Before a workout, consider having nuts like almonds, yogurt in a shake, or hard boiled eggs. You can also make your own granola bars or trail mix, or you can have a wheat muffin with peanut butter or eggs in a pita before you head to the gym.

Make Your Own Favorite Foods

As you get further along in the DASH diet and you start combining foods to make your own healthy recipes, you may find that you want to make your own great snacks, such as granola bars.

You can incorporate things like molasses and honey into them. You can also fill them with lots of good nuts and seeds to give you the nutrients and minerals that you need and to fuel yourself during a workout.

Shakes And Protein

You can also make your own protein shakes to give you the fuel you will need for a workout. Try having a shake with yogurt, strawberries, bananas, cucumbers, broccoli, peppers, and anything else with fiber for fuel.

This will also aid in digestion, so you won't have to worry about having problems with constipation. If, on the other hand, you have a problem with loose bowels, then make your protein shakes a little bit milder; have something like a mango protein shake with watermelon, a cantaloupe shake with strawberries, or a banana, and limit your greens until you finish your workout at the gym. Adding veggies to a shake is about balance for your digestion, and you will know when you need to add more green!

Curb Cravings

If you have cravings during your workout or even at lunchtime, a small snack, such as a bag of almonds or a few pieces of low-fat cheese, can work wonders. You can also have a nice, healthy salad at lunchtime, with lettuce, tomatoes, tuna salad, and red onions in it. You can use a low-fat pita to hold it. This meal will give you enough protein to get through lunch and the workout.

Work On Building Muscle

Make sure you use a good cardiovascular workout that utilizes the treadmill, elliptical, or stair master. You also want to ensure that you start building muscle because doing so burns fat, which helps you lose weight. Keep in mind that gaining muscle may initially cause you to appear like you're gaining weight.

Workouts are also about longevity. You want to ensure you're combining your food with a consistent workout regimen. You don't want to try to burn as many calories as you can and then come back the next day and do the same thing; you will quickly burn yourself out, and you don't want to do that. Work out and train consistently, and in the long run, your body will feel better and you will be able to maintain optimal health. Be sure to stretch and drink a lot of water before, during, and after your workouts.

Burning More Calories

A lot of people switch over to the DASH diet because they want to learn how to eat healthy and exercise for life. When you watch certain shows about weight loss, they may show people in the gym who try to burn 6,000 calories a day. These shows let you see people who drop ten pounds a week, and that's not healthy. Not only does it lead to stress fractures, but you can lose so much salt that you end up in the hospital. That is not your goal. You want to work on a consistent plan. If you want to burn a pound in a week, you will have to burn 3,500 calories per week to lose that pound.

This kind of weight loss can also be achieved by taking in fewer calories per week. You want to find a good balance between your workouts and your diet. Try to incorporate protein shakes into your workouts. Include things like bananas and yogurt that have potassium. Incorporating a lot of calcium into your diet, and give your body enough fuel to exercise.

The Dangers Of Mercury

Be careful with having a lot of fish in your diet. You may think having tuna every day at lunchtime will help you lose weight, but you have to be very careful with your mercury intake. Try to have no more than the equivalent of two cans of tuna per week. Mercury can damage the kidneys, and you don't want to have to worry about this.

CHAPTER 3
LOWERING BLOOD PRESSURE: FOODS AND MINERALS THAT HELP

If you've ever had to wear a monitor to keep track of your blood pressure, or if you've ever had to take blood pressure medicine, then you know that one of the best things you can do is lower your blood pressure naturally.

There are a few key ways to do this, which you should consider doing if you don't want to be on blood pressure medicine for the rest of your life. This medicine may lower your blood pressure and heart rate, but it could also have adverse effects such as sluggishness. It would be best if you didn't have to take any blood pressure medication.

Keep in mind that with the DASH diet, there are certain foods that will naturally lower your blood pressure. Foods that are rich in potassium, for example, and foods such as potatoes, sweet potatoes, and even bananas help with your pressure. Other foods that can help include ginger, as ginger is anti-inflammatory.

Incorporate foods that are rich in vitamins and minerals into your diet. This way you're actually targeting a homeopathic way of changing your lifestyle by changing your eating habits. Also include magnesium and potassium, which can fuel your body and combat various diseases and illnesses.

Consult A Physician

If you're on blood pressure medication, check with your doctor to discuss coming off of it. If your pressure is usually 180 over 100, taking your blood pressure medicine may lower it to a healthy 120 over 80. When you start eating a diet, your blood pressure may drop even lower—too low, like to 90 over 60! You could have trouble standing up and may get dizzy, and you definitely don't want that.

Your doctor may lower the blood pressure medicine as you are on the diet to avoid this problem. You can also ask your doctor about investing in a blood pressure cuff so you can keep track of your blood pressure at home. Don't ever stop a blood pressure medication suddenly, and don't stop it on your own. You have to consult with a doctor, as sudden changes can be life-threatening.

Daily Intake

If you're doing a regular DASH diet, you want to try to consume about 2,200 to 2,300 milligrams of sodium every day. For a low-salt DASH diet, try to keep it down to about 1,500 milligrams of salt per day. This would be useful if you are worried about your health, are over the age of fifty, or have high blood pressure, a heart condition, hypertension, diabetes, or kidney disorders.

On the DASH diet, ideally you want to consume about 2,000 calories per day.

This will include all sorts of great nutritional products, such as beans, poultry, fish, and some red meat—in moderation. You can still have sweets and low-fat products in small quantities. So, let's take a look at the breakdown.

Cereal, Pasta, And Bread

Ideally you want to have about six to eight servings per day. You can have cereal for breakfast time, pasta for lunch with tuna salad, and rice with dinner. Also keep in mind that you're going to make substitutions, such as whole wheat bread or 100% whole grain bread instead of white bread, brown rice instead of white rice, and wheat pasta instead of regular pasta.

Carrots, Broccoli And Green Leafy Vegetables

You generally want to stick to about four to five servings of veggies each day. try to incorporate various veggies into each meal. At breakfast time, you may have carrots and celery in a shake; when you make eggs, you may add onions and green peppers.

At lunchtime, you want to always incorporate a salad, whether it's a fruit salad or a regular salad made with mixed greens and lots of veggies. At dinnertime, try to have a salad and a hearty, leafy green vegetable like kale or spinach. Don't buy canned vegetables, which can have a lot of salt in them. Instead, look for frozen or fresh.

High Mineral Content

Your vegetables should also be rich in iron, zinc, magnesium, potassium, and other minerals and nutrients. Make sure you target foods like kale, spinach, sweet potatoes, broccoli, squash, zucchini, tomatoes, peas, green beans, eggplant, red onions, garlic, and ginger, which are very heart-healthy.

Strawberries, Bananas, Avocados, And More

Have at least four to five servings of fruit each day. The purpose of this is to ensure that as you ingest fiber; it helps with digestion. Part of the DASH diet is about having high protein, and the fiber will help to ensure that you're able to digest your food more easily. Another benefit is that you're also ingesting a lot of vitamins and nutrients that your body needs.

Milk And Yogurt

If you're going to have dairy products in your diet, such as milk or yogurt, you want to try to have at least three servings per day. This can be incorporated into things such as low-fat and low-sodium cheese, yogurt, and milk. You can have milk with cereal. Your yogurt can go into a parfait, smoothie, or protein shake, and cheese can be an afternoon snack.

Seafood, Poultry And Red Meat

Have six servings of meat each day. You can have low-sodium bacon in the morning. You can have turkey, chicken, or tuna fish at lunchtime, or mix them up in a healthy salad or pita wrap. Dinner can be any assortment of meats such as salmon, tilapia, red meat like ground beef, or steak in moderation, depending on your cholesterol. Meats are a good source of protein and include iron and zinc as well as vitamin B.

Peanuts, Almonds, And Sunflower Seeds

You want to ensure that you have nuts, beans, and seeds in your diet—at least four to five servings each week. Make sure you don't have a lot of high-fat nuts like pistachios. If you happen to be a vegetarian, you will find that your nut and seed consumption incorporated with soy-based products can work well in the DASH diet. You can also incorporate things like tofu into a healthy salad that has lots of veggies and nuts in it.

Some foods to consider are walnuts, almonds, pecans, peanuts, and even pine nuts in moderation. Beans such as edamame, lentils, black beans, navy beans, red beans, pinto beans, and chickpeas are rich in fiber and have a lot of minerals and nutrients in them. When you start making your own soups and dips, like hummus, you can really come up with great recipes.

Sugar And Your Sweet Tooth

Your sweet tooth may be calling, but try to limit your sugar intake. Eventually you'll be able to fight off the sugar cravings. Don't switch over to diet sodas because they are just as bad for you, and don't necessarily switch over to artificial sweeteners which can also be just as bad or even worse; try to cut down on the amount of real sugar that you use.

You can look for sugar-free versions of different things like hard candies, cookies, and even sorbets and ice creams. If you are having trouble finding these, consider making your own. It's not that difficult to make your own sorbet, and you may actually find that you enjoy it more as you experiment with different flavors.

Fatty Foods And Oil-Based Products

Try to limit your fatty foods to two to three servings each day. Consume good fats and not bad fats. Good fats are saturated; bad fats are trans fats. Trans fats are normally found in fried food, so don't fry your food. You can bake everything instead. If you want something like fried chicken, there are several ways to bake it that make it taste better—try dipping the chicken in a nice batter and adding Panko bread crumbs for extra crunch!

To ensure that you get enough saturated fat but you don't overdo it, try to limit how much butter, cheese, cream, and eggs you consume. Use real butter instead of margarine, and simply use less of it. For any salad dressings that you would use, check the salt and fat contents so you don't have too much of either one.

CHAPTER 4
ADJUSTMENTS: TRACKING CHANGES AND MAKING DAILY ADJUSTMENTS

If you're working on the DASH diet, you want to keep in mind that there are going to be daily adjustments that you have to make. For example, you may be out with friends and family and you're tempted to order those greasy nachos or that fried food. You have to be strong and remember that on the DASH diet, you can have those same great foods but in a healthier version.

With your diet adjustments, your way of cooking will be about adding more nutrients and ensuring you have foods with less salt in them. The problem is, though, it's hard when you're not at home because sometimes you're hungry and you just don't know what to eat. That's where the DASH diet comes in.

Making Substitutions

As you start to look at your daily intake of food, you're going to have to make adjustments. For example, if you are out and you go for lunch with friends, maybe there are healthy alternatives that you can find at a restaurant. You could have a buffet-style salad where you can build your own salad, or maybe you can order a piece of grilled chicken with lots of steamed veggies.

Modify Any Menu

Sometimes, though, you may find that there are no healthy alternatives in an area you go to with friends and family. They may pick the fast food joint, or the restaurant with really unhealthy options. That's where you have to be very careful with what you eat. You may have to ask for specific things that you can have, like sliced tomatoes, lettuce, and tuna salad with no salt, and specify how you want it to be delivered.

For example, instead of a tuna salad on toasted bread with grilled cheese, get it on a pita without the grilled cheese. The cheese won't be low-fat, and the bread may be white bread.

Don't Be Afraid To Ask For Healthier Options

Also be sure to ask for something like a low-fat yogurt and mixed fruit. When eating out with friends or family, you may have trouble finding something that you can have. Eat differently than you normally would so that you consume less sodium. Keep in mind that a majority of fried foods are high in salt.

Plan Ahead

You can carry food with you. For example, if you know that you're going to be out for a long day, take a snack with you. Carry almonds in your bag, as almonds are light and also filling. Or think about carrying a little stick of low-fat cheese. Also think about something like grape tomatoes that you can take with you on the go.

As you make small adjustments to your snacks, you're also going to want to ensure that you incorporate this into all of your meals. Additionally, encourage your family to eat the same healthy diet so they can fight illnesses and diseases like you're doing.

Making Meal Adjustments

Let's target different areas that have to be adjusted. Maybe you're not used to having breakfast because you don't have time to make it. You can always carry packets of oatmeal with you. Preferably, you want to look at something like steel-cut oats, which have lower salt and more vitamins, nutrients, and minerals.

Or you could grab a protein shake, which is fast. Make it the night before and leave it in the blender in the refrigerator, and in the morning, have your shake and go. In your shake, you could combine granola, yogurt, and a lot of fruit and baby spinach; that way, you will be loading up on healthy nutrition.

Breakfast On The Go

Another option is having hard boiled eggs for breakfast. You can carry these to work with you because they're easy to transport. In traffic on your way to work, you can have something healthy like a protein shake to hold you over until you get to the office.

Healthy Snacks

When you buy your snacks, buy lots of healthy alternative such as grape tomatoes, edamame, celery sticks, and baby carrots, that way you have little things that you can graze on when you want to have a light snack.

If you want something sweet, go for strawberries or even cherries.

Because you're seeking out healthy alternatives, you're always going to keep something on hand that can serve as a light and healthy snack. If it's hard to fight these cravings, consider having something like home-made baked potato chips that you slice thin and bake in the oven.

You could also have nuts that you roast in a pan. You can quickly make this with almonds, sunflower seeds, and peanuts. Just throw everything in and sauté it lightly. It only takes a few minutes. You can even have it over yogurt for added benefit, but save some for your salad later!

Lunch At Work

As you are at work, it may be hard to find good, healthy options. Try to incorporate chicken, turkey, tuna fish, or salmon into your lunch. For other meals at lunchtime, you can try grilled chicken or oven-roasted turkey breast. Do not buy deli meat turkey or meat that is sold pre-packaged. These are usually extremely high in salt and nitrates. Only seek out the oven-roasted versions to reduce salt consumption.

You can also have multigrain breads with your meat: nut breads, whole wheat bread, or wheat pitas. Look for the low-carb alternatives. If you can have a salad at work each day, that would be great; add more healthy veggies beyond the basic lettuce and tomatoes such as green peppers, red peppers, cucumber, radishes, shredded carrots, celery, onions, red onions, corn, green beans, and broccoli.

As you can see, by incorporating more sources of fiber, protein, and nutrient-rich foods into your lunch, you're fueling your body, giving it what it needs, and not consuming high-salt foods.

Dinner

A lot of restaurants have dishes that might look healthy, but they are really loaded with a lot of salt and saturated fats. For example, you have to be careful with some restaurant chains out there.

Look for the calorie breakdown on their menus so you can see which selections are low in salt. Also make sure that you're sticking with your diet by getting things such as a piece of grilled chicken or a piece of grilled salmon and a healthy salad or mixed vegetables with it.

TIP: Want to look like you're not even on a diet? If you know to which restaurant you're going, check out their menu online ahead of time. That way when they ask you for your order, you won't sound awkward or like you've been put on the spot!

Ordering Food At Venues

For the times that you may want to go out to a movie or to a baseball game, for example, you don't want anything that is processed or frozen. Most of the available foods, such as hot dogs, French fries, and popcorn, will be high in salt.

It would be better for you to bring something healthy from home such as your cheese, grape tomatoes, celery, or carrots. Avoid eating something that's going to increase your blood pressure. If you can't take food with you, get peanuts in the shells or fries with no salt..

TIP: If you ever find that your feet are starting to swell, ask yourself what it was that you ate that day. Sometimes there are hidden salts in things like spaghetti sauce, barbecue sauce, and salad dressing. With a low-salt diet, you'll be able to tell as soon as you have something that has a lot of salt because you might be retaining water the next day!

Snacks You Make Yourself

People who are used to snacking on chips may find it hard to start with the DASH diet because they're so used to having the salt. An alternative is something like trail mix or granola mix that you make yourself. Even some new cereals now have high protein levels in them. Just make sure they are low in salt.

Ready-To-Go Snacks

Keep your granola in little baggies, and always take some with you. You should always have ready-to-go foods in your refrigerator, like cut-up apples, hard boiled eggs, and other foods you can take with you. You can also buy little Jell-O cups; make sure they are sugar-free and they can travel well. Don't forget the spoon!

Chapter 5
Meal Plans: Sample Diets, Tips and Pointers

How To Start The DASH Diet: A Sample Menu

When you start the DASH diet, you're going to want to incorporate a few things that you might not think about all the time. This is going to take some time to get used to. Maybe you are used to grabbing a bagel with cream cheese for breakfast, or you're used to just getting a burger on the go. With the DASH diet, you're going to think about different ways that you can incorporate fresh food into your meal plans. The first place you want to begin is in the grocery aisle.

Better Grocery Shopping

Be sure that you buy healthy foods. A good place to start with is your juice aisle. Yes, you will be able to have your favorite juices. You should buy juices like:

- Low-sodium tomato juice
- Sugar-free cranberry juice
- Orange juice
- Apple juice

Produce

Next, when you buy your actual foods, you want to look for things in your produce aisle such as lettuce, tomatoes, bell peppers, grape tomatoes, regular tomatoes, carrots, and baby carrots.

Snacks

Be sure to buy things that you will enjoy, such as sugar-free Jell-O, which can be fillers and don't have high calories. Also look for low-fat cottage cheese, cranberries, dried fruit, and healthy nuts like peanuts in the shells, cashews, pistachios, pecans, walnuts, and almonds.

Meat And Seafood

Next, you want to look for meat that you're going to be making fresh, so look for things like oven-roasted turkey, chicken breasts, whole chickens, legs and thighs that you can bake, and fish like tilapia, salmon, or flounder. Don't limit yourself with the meat and seafood; you can make great salads with shrimp or shrimp and grilled steak. While you don't want to have a lot of red meat, you can have beef stew, roast beef, and pot roast, as these will likely have you tossing a lot of veggies into the mix.

Sauces And Dressings

Look at your dressings and any sauces that you would use on them. If you make a sauce for spaghetti, try to make it one that is fresh from tomatoes or tomato paste as opposed to one that is a pre-made spaghetti sauce in a can, as these tend to have a lot of salt in them. If you do have to go with a high-salt kind, you can always dilute the sauce with a little water.

PHASE 1

This is the weight loss phase of the DASH diet, and we've included a sample menu to show you all the great options you can enjoy!

Breakfast

A sample breakfast might include egg whites, scrambled eggs or egg beaters, and low-salt juice.

Morning Snacks

A morning snack might be something like grape tomatoes, celery sticks, or baby carrots. You could also include a little piece of low-fat cheese or hard boiled eggs, which are nice sources of protein.

Lunch

For lunch, look for something like smoked turkey, oven-roasted turkey, or chicken that's been grilled. Have it with or in a salad, and consider your sugar-free Jell-O for a light dessert or filler. Also consider a light snack like popcorn with no butter or salt that you make at home

Afternoon Snacks

A snack in the afternoon could be something like a handful of almonds and a few carrots, or you can have the Jell-O if you didn't have to earlier in the day.

Dinner

When you get to dinner, you may want to think about something like your
oven-roasted chicken or turkey and a side of mixed vegetables, or you could have a salad with a very light dressing. You can make your own vinaigrette or use a light olive oil as a dressing.

Dessert

For your dessert, maybe have Jell-O, or have a little piece of cheese and tomatoes. If you really want something sweet, have a few strawberries and some almonds.

As you reprogram your brain to eat real foods, you will notice that everything that you added was healthy, protein-rich, and high in nutrients and minerals, such as veggies, fruit, and dairy.

PHASE 2

As you go into Phase 2, this is where you're going to start to add more healthy foods. Keep in mind that this phase is for when you've achieved your actual weight loss and are now targeting higher proteins, higher fiber, lower fat, and lower salt.

Breakfast

For breakfast, consider having scrambled eggs or hard boiled eggs. You can also have a little bit of fruit, like a mixed fruit cup or a blend of strawberries and bananas. You can have orange juice, coffee or hot chocolate.

Morning Snack

For a morning snack, consider having almonds and low-fat yogurt. This can help ensure that you curb any cravings. The almonds also serve as a small way to burn fat.

Lunch

At lunchtime, you can make your own turkey, chicken, or tuna wrap. You can use lettuce, a pita, or a tortilla shell, and then add in healthy veggies like onions and peppers if you would like. Fill it with tomatoes and lettuce, roll it up, and enjoy!

Afternoon Snack

For your afternoon snack, you can have a little more protein, like a handful of nuts again. You can have yogurt, a fruit cup, or Jell-O. Try having peanuts in the shells; you'll actually eat less this way.

Dinner

For dinner, make something hearty like grilled chicken parmesan. Serve it with a red sauce, and add a little low-fat cheese to it. You could also add squash, zucchini, and other vegetables to your sauce to make it rich. Have a big side salad with that and you may not even want dessert!

Dessert

If you still have room for dessert, consider having strawberries, almonds, or a yogurt parfait.

As you see from the diet, you're incorporating homemade foods, avoiding fried and salted foods, and consuming foods that are rich in nutrients and minerals. This can help lower your blood pressure and keep it low. Ultimately, your weight loss and diet changes are about setting goals and achieving them one step at a time.

Because I know that the DASH diet is something that you could accomplish successfully over time, it's just a matter of changing your thinking. That's why I've put together a few tips that can help you reprogram your mind and reassess your eating habits.

Say No To Processed Foods

When you go through your cabinets, get rid of frozen, processed, or high-salt foods. That means frozen pizzas, frozen TV dinners, frozen chicken nuggets, frozen French fries, or anything that is processed should be thrown out. Fill your freezer with healthy options like frozen fruit, veggies, and fresh meat. Always think less salt. The DASH diet is going to help you lower your salt intake, and this can help lower your blood pressure. But that means you're going to have to do your homework as well.

Read The Labels

Look at the salt content of whatever it is that you're eating. For example, a bag of chips may have 250 milligrams of salt. Can you find one that's only 60 to 80 milligrams of salt? You want to eat healthy and be consistent about it as much as you can.

Restock The Shelves

Be sure to restock the shelves with the foods that you will be eating in the diet. Make a list of all the new goodies that you're going to pick up at the store, such as yogurt, mixed nuts, veggies, and fruit. The one thing that causes people to fall away from a diet is when they say, "Oh, I can't find anything to eat." That's not true. You just don't know what to eat—yet. That's why you have to make sure you have things that you can have on the diet. It will be quite a lot, so experiment!

Coming Up With New Recipes

Your new diet and new way of looking at food will have you enjoying a lot of great, new dishes. However, you may find that you feel like you're just having the same thing every day. So, as you work on your diet plan, focus on new ways to eat healthy and on new recipes that can be used with the DASH diet. Don't be afraid to put that fruit in the oven and dry it out for a tasty treat. Don't be afraid to have peanuts in the shells. Don't be afraid to bake kale or make your own granola bars. That's the fun of a new diet: making it your own!

Time To Adjust

Because the concept is new, it will take time to adjust. Give yourself time and you'll see how the benefits pay off down the road. Look for ways that you can use the DASH diet to make healthier versions of the foods you may start to miss.

Revamp Fries And Pizza

For example, if you liked having pizza, whether it was frozen or you ordered it, you can still have it as a better version. Try experimenting with a pita, fresh tomatoes, and low-fat and low-salt cheese. Maybe you were used to those greasy French fries. Well, you can still have them; just ensure that you're utilizing all fresh ingredients, like fresh-cut white potatoes or sweet potatoes. That way you can make sure that you're getting the nutrients your body needs.

CONCLUSION

The goal as you adjust to the DASH diet is to work on the ways you can lower salt, adjust to new foods, and substitute salty, processed, and fried foods with fresh foods. These new foods are better for you and safer for your body. That's the main goal of the diet—to ingest food that your body will benefit from and will put to good use. You don't want to have your body loaded with salt, because then you're causing your heart to work harder and making your blood pressure skyrocket.

The next step in making the DASH diet work is having a mineral-rich diet with lots of nutrients and vitamins. As you are feeding your body the proper foods, not only will it work more productively for you, but you'll see your skin has a healthier glow to it, you'll feel rejuvenated, you'll lose weight, and you'll be able to fight off all those nasty diseases and illnesses that you couldn't before.

Don't see the DASH diet as a way for a quick fix. See it as a move that will allow you to eat healthy for life. People are learning that not only are they living healthier lives, but they have a bounce-back like they never did before! That's what you should have too. Each day should be an empowered one; have the healthy eating habits that will fuel your body from the time you get up to when you go to bed each night. You should also incorporate the DASH diet into what you feed your family because these healthy options will benefit them as well!

Did you Like "The DASH Diet for Weight Loss"?

Before you go, I'd like to say "thank you so much" for purchasing my book.

I know you could have picked from dozens of books on this subject, but you took a chance with mine and I'm truly grateful for that.

So once again, a big thanks for downloading this book and reading all the way to the end, I truly appreciate it.

Now I'd like to ask for a small favor if you don't mind . . .

Would you be so kind as to take a minute of your time and leave a review for this book on Amazon.

This feedback will help me continue to write the kind of books that help you get results. And if you loved it then please feel free to let me know! :)